Healing
is Easy

By
Stacy Adams

TABLE OF CONTENTS

INTRODUCTION

Have you ever wondered if healing is for today or why some people are healed and some remain sick or die? Is it God's will to heal me? Is it God's timing?

It is God's will that we are healed. Healing is for now, not in the distant future. God has made a way for healing and it is not complicated.

This book is a quick reference to healing scriptures and a guide to healing. My suggestion is to read through the book more than once, really meditating on the scriptures.

As you read this book, pray the Holy Spirit will open your eyes and heart to the truths of God's word. If you have any preconceived ideas, opinions or prejudices against healing, set them aside. If you are truly seeking the truth, you will find it.

2 Timothy 3:16-17 16 All Scripture *is* given by inspiration of God, and *is* profitable for doctrine, for reproof, for correction, for [a]instruction in righteousness, 17 that the man of God may be complete, thoroughly equipped for every good work.

Jeremiah 33:3 3 'Call to Me, and I will answer you, and show you great and [a]mighty things, which you do not know.'

John 8:32 32 And you shall know the truth, and the truth shall make you free."

John 8:36 36 Therefore if the Son makes you free, you shall be free indeed.

FIRST THINGS FIRST

Once, I read a warning about half truths. It said, "Be aware of the half-truth, you may have gotten hold of the wrong half."

Now, the half-truth in many cases may, or may not cause trouble in your life. However, if you do not know the truth about Jesus, or only know the half-truth, it will cause an eternity of trouble for you.

John 14:6 6 Jesus said to him, "I am the way, the truth, and the life. No one comes to the Father except through Me.~ Jesus Christ

GOOD NEWS (The Best You Can Ever Hear)
If you do not know Jesus personally, I would like to introduce Him to you. Jesus is the best friend you can ever have, and He will never let you down.

RECOGNIZE JESUS HAS A PLAN FOR YOU AND LOVES YOU

Jeremiah 29:11 11 For I know the thoughts that I think toward you, says the Lord, thoughts of peace and not of evil, to give you a future and a hope.

SIN SEPARATES PEOPLE FROM GOD

Romans 3:23 23 **for all have sinned and fall short of the glory of God,**

Romans 6:23 23 **For the wages of sin** *is* **death, but the** [a]**gift of God** *is* **eternal life in Christ Jesus our Lord.**

The bible says everyone is a sinner. Anything we do to work toward our right standing with God is not enough to save us, that's why Jesus came.

GOD'S SOLUTION

Romans 5:8 8 **But God demonstrates His own love toward us, in that while we were still sinners, Christ died for us.**

1 John 2:2 2 **And He Himself is the propitiation** *(Atoning Sacrifice)* **for our sins, and not for ours only but also for the whole world.**

John 3:16-17 16 **For God so loved the world that He gave His only begotten Son, that whoever believes in Him should not perish but have everlasting life.** 17 **For God did not send His Son into the world to condemn the world, but that the world through Him might be saved.**

Jesus is the payment for our sins. Sins cannot be paid off any other way. Good works, being a good person, giving money to church, church attendance or any other deed we do to get in good standing with God is never enough. Only Jesus is enough.

GOD'S FREE LOVE GIFT TO YOU

Ephesians 2:8-9 8 For by grace you have been saved through faith, and that not of yourselves; *it is* the gift of God, 9 not of works, lest anyone should boast.

Salvation is a gift from God. Just believing God exists is not enough to be saved. We must accept the gift from God by believing, receiving and trusting in God. Put your full faith and trust in Jesus' sacrifice for your salvation.

RECEIVE JESUS AS YOUR SAVIOR

Romans 10:9-13 9 that if you confess with your mouth the Lord Jesus and believe in your heart that God has raised Him from the dead, you will be saved. 10 For

with the heart one believes unto righteousness, and with the mouth confession is made unto salvation. 11 For the Scripture says, "Whoever believes on Him will not be put to shame." 12 For there is no distinction between Jew and Greek, for the same Lord over all is rich to all who call upon Him. 13 For "whoever calls on the name of the LORD shall be saved."

It is not enough to know about Jesus, you must believe with your heart and know Him personally. Everyone is a sinner and needs a Savior. Accept what Jesus has done for you. Salvation is a gift that is received by faith. Put your full trust in Jesus for your salvation. The moment you believe the gospel, you receive Jesus as your Lord and Savior; you are born again.

To confess with your mouth, you can pray something like this: Jesus, I know that I am a sinner and I need your forgiveness. I believe you died in my place and rose again, paying for my sins. I accept your gift of salvation and ask you to come into my heart and be my Lord and Savior. Amen

If you have accepted Jesus as your Lord and Savior, look for a bible believing church to attend, read your bible asking the Holy Spirit to teach you and talk to Jesus every day. Jesus is alive, and He wants you to be blessed in everything you do.

CHAPTER 1
God's Will for Healing

~

Being sick and going through trials can be tough and sometimes it may seem like we are all alone. Have you ever wondered if God is there? If He caused your situation? Have you wondered if He hears you? If He cares what is happening to you? And if He really cares, why isn't He doing anything?

Jesus always preached the gospel of the Kingdom of God which includes not only salvation, but healing and deliverance to those who believe. He did not separate salvation and healing, the two always went hand in hand. Today, many only preach salvation, leaving healing as a separate gift only for some. We must remember Jesus' sacrifice was a completed work encompassing our healing, deliverance and saving grace.

**Psalm 145:9 9 The Lord *is* good to all,
And His tender mercies *are* over all His works.**

We need to know that God is a good God and that He wants the best for us in every situation. We must establish this truth in our hearts.

When it comes to getting any prayer answered, including healing, we must decide who we are going to believe. Who are you going to believe: the doctor, the devil, your body or God?

The doctor: The doctor gives medical answers to sickness and disease. The doctor does his or her best to educate the patient on the disease, sometimes giving the worst-case scenario just in case everything goes wrong. Perhaps the doctor prescribes medications to alleviate the symptoms but not heal the sickness.

The devil: Yes, he is real. Yes, he is a liar. Yes, he will do everything in his power to get us to believe the lie of sickness, disease and death. The devil will attempt to get us to believe God has placed the illness on us or God isn't going to heal us. The bible warns us not to be ignorant of the devil's ways.

Our body: Our bodies can speak to us also. Pain, weakness, discomfort, feelings of discouragement can keep us stuck in sickness if our body is our focus. Our bodies cannot be the "boss" when it comes to getting healed. I'm not saying that what our bodies experience isn't real, I'm saying that God is greater. We must resist the symptoms and focus on God.

God: God is the answer to our healing. Jesus paid the price for every sickness and disease just as He paid the price for sins. Jesus is the one we want to align our belief system with if we want to see healing.

THE QUESTION: Do you believe it is ALWAYS God's will to heal EVERY person, EVERY time?

THE ANSWER: The answer is a confident YES! God says His promises are Yes and Amen.

If we have any other answer than yes or waiver between yes and no, we have positioned ourselves in a place of doubt and unbelief.

When we are ignorant of how something works, it is difficult to get positive results.

Example: You get a brand-new lawn mower. You can start the engine but do not know how to engage the mower. At this point, you will not be able to cut your grass until you figure out how to engage the mower.

Your neighbor comes over to help you. He says to get your tools and let's remove the tires to get the blades closer to the ground. The neighbor tells you it will be more difficult to drive but at least the blades are down.

If you follow your neighbor's instructions, you will not get the lawn mower to cut the grass because the mower will not function properly. The entire time it was as simple as pulling a lever to engage the mower. But if you lack that piece of vital information, you are stuck.

Wrong information, wrong teaching and wrong thinking will keep us stuck. Just like the lawnmower, the same happens with healing. We can be stuck until we understand how it works. Jesus made healing simple and man has complicated it.

Many people talk about God as a good, good Father. Some call him Daddy, yet believe He places sickness on us or doesn't want everyone healed. I don't know any father or daddy that loves their children and would want them sick or suffering. "Here honey, let me give you cancer and teach you a lesson." None of us want a loved one or a child sick or suffering. How much more does God want to give us GOOD gifts (Matthew 7:11)? God is love and only He is good. He certainly wants us well.

God loves us and He loves our children more than we could ever love someone. We are smart enough to know sickness is bad and do not want our children sick or want to be sick ourselves.

God can turn any situation around and give us a testimony but this doesn't mean He caused the negative situation. He is not the problem and the answer, He is ONLY the answer.

I have listened to people who believe God gave them an illness so they can minister to others. Jesus ministered to others without being sick, and so can we. Sickness does not glorify God, healing does. People can learn lessons from anything, good or bad, but again, it does not mean God caused the sickness or the negative situation.

We can have some ridiculous thoughts at times. If we truly believe that God does not want everyone well or that He places sickness on us to teach us a lesson, we should not be seeking healing or seeking to be well. We should stop going to the doctor, stop taking medication, stop praying for the sick, and stop working against God. We should stay sick and learn the whole lesson. We should pray things like, "God if it is your will to heal her, heal her. If it is not your will, just kill her." Or "Lord, just let him continue to suffer. Amen." Most people would not pray "just kill her" or "let him continue to suffer", but that is in essence what we are saying when we pray like this. If we do not know God's will, how will we know what to pray?

Internally we know that it's God's will to heal or we would not seek out healing. God created the body to heal itself. If He didn't want us well, He would not have created us this way. When we believe contrary to God's word, healing is blocked.

Hosea 4:6 6 My people are destroyed for lack of knowledge. Because you have rejected knowledge, I also will reject you from being priest for Me; Because you have forgotten the law of your God, I also will forget your children.

Hosea 4:6 says God's people are destroyed for lack of knowledge. I know of people who want to be healed but never study healing and do not have a scripture to stand on in faith. We must put some effort into our relationship with God to know His benefits and His character. God is love!

Proverbs 4:7 7 Wisdom *is* the principal thing; *Therefore* get wisdom. And in all your getting, get understanding.

Too often when we do not understand something in God's word, we do not seek His wisdom, we seek man's understanding. To get God's results we need God's wisdom. We cannot take man's teaching and our negative experiences and place them above God's word and expect we will get God's results. We must do things God's way to get God's results.

We must understand without question or doubt that it is God's will for everyone to be well.

3 John 2 2 Beloved, I pray that you may prosper in all things and be in health, just as your soul prospers.

John 10:10 10 The thief does not come except to steal, and to kill, and to destroy. I have come that they may have life, and that they may have *it* more abundantly.

Sickness and disease do not fall into the category of abundant life. Sickness robs our energy, time, joy, finances and peace. Sickness can kill us. Sickness is from the enemy.

**Matthew 6:9-13 9 In this manner, therefore, pray: Our Father in heaven, Hallowed be Your name.
10 Your kingdom come. Your will be done On earth as *it is* in heaven. 11 Give us this day our daily bread. 12 And forgive us our debts, As we forgive our debtors. 13 And do not lead us into temptation,
But deliver us from the evil one. [a]For Yours is the kingdom and the power and the glory forever. Amen.**

God's Kingdom lives in those who believe.

His will be done on earth as it is in heaven says it all. There is NO sickness in heaven.

Healing is the children's bread (Mark 7:25-30).

Sickness is a temptation that must be resisted just like any other temptation.

Forgiveness toward others is essential. Unforgiveness toward others affects our bodies negatively.

Exodus 15:26 26 and said, "If you diligently heed the voice of the Lᴏʀᴅ your God and do what is right in His sight, give ear to His commandments and keep all His statutes, I will put none of the diseases on you which I have brought on the Egyptians. For I *am* the Lᴏʀᴅ who heals you."

Psalm 103:2-5 2 Bless the Lᴏʀᴅ, O my soul, And forget not all His benefits: 3 Who forgives all your iniquities, Who heals all your diseases, 4 Who redeems your life from destruction, Who crowns you with lovingkindness and tender mercies, 5 Who satisfies your mouth with good *things, So that* your youth is renewed like the eagle's.

1 Peter 2:24 24 who Himself bore our sins in His own body on the tree, that we, having died to sins, might live for righteousness—by whose [a]stripes you were healed.

Matthew 8:16-17 16 When evening had come, they brought to Him many who were demon-possessed. And He cast out the spirits with a word, and healed all who were sick, 17 that it might be fulfilled which was spoken by Isaiah the prophet, saying:

"He Himself took our infirmities
And bore *our* sicknesses."

Sickness and disease are a result of sin and are listed as curses in Deuteronomy 28. Galatians chapter 3 says that Jesus redeemed us from the curse. Jesus paid the price, therefore, we do not need to live under the curse. We do not need to accept sickness. Sickness belongs to the devil, not us.

Galatians 3:13 13 Christ has redeemed us from the curse of the law, having become a curse for us (for it is written, "Cursed *is* everyone who hangs on a tree"),

Jeremiah 29:11-13 11 For I know the thoughts that I think toward you, says the Lord**, thoughts of peace and not of evil, to give you a future and a hope. 12 Then you will call upon Me and go and pray to Me, and I will listen to you. 13 And you will seek Me and find *Me,* when you search for Me with all your heart.**

Remember that the Lord has good plans for us. We must stand firm on God's word where healing is concerned. It is God's will for all to be healed every single time; no exceptions. Settle this in your heart so healing can begin to flow through you. Think about how much Jesus loves you! He thinks you are wonderful and would do anything to help you. He calls you blessed.

Wrong thinking and wrong believing block the flow of God's healing. Think of it as a clogged pipe or a dirty air filter. When things are clogged, they do not work right.

Water will not flow freely through the pipes until the clog is removed. Air cannot flow freely through a dirty air filter. The same is true for God's healing power to flow, we must unclog our hearts and get rid of wrong thinking and wrong believing to allow God's healing to flow through our bodies.

I had a dream of a man strapped into a high-back wheelchair because he was paralyzed from the neck down. His head and arms were strapped down to the chair, he was completely immobile. Jesus walked into the room and His presence was overwhelming. Every single strap broke loose from the wheelchair and the man was instantly healed. Then Jesus said, "Tell my people to stop trying to carry the burdens I've already carried."

Sickness is not our burden to bear, Christ already bore it. Our portion is healing.

CHAPTER 2

Questions About Healing

~

There are a lot of opinions and questions about healing in the church. God's opinion is the only opinion we should care about.

Does God still heal today?

If God heals, why am I still sick?

Why does God heal some and not others?

Is it God's will for everyone to be healed?

What about Paul's thorn?

Yes, God still heals today. If we are going to see healing manifest when we pray, we must tear down strongholds of wrong thinking. If we are seeking healing, we cannot be seeking scriptures or experiences that would seem to justify illness. We cannot be seeking and studying information contrary to God's word. There are teachings in churches that are taught as truth but are in fact just religious teachings, man's traditions, not based on the truth of God's word. We need to go back to the word of God for all truth.

Do not look to negative experiences that contradict God's word, such as praying for someone to be healed and they die. This could look as though it must not have been God's will for the person to be healed. This is not the case. The problem is not on God's end, it is on ours. Perhaps the person we prayed for did not receive the healing or want to be healed. I've had people say they don't want to be prayed for to be healed because they just want to go to heaven. If that is the case, my prayer would not override their will and they wouldn't be healed.

Other experiences: Perhaps we prayed a prayer of begging God verses commanding the sickness. Maybe we did not expect the person to be healed. There can be a lot of varying factors on our end. That's why it is important we get our belief system aligned with God's word.

One of God's names is Jehovah-Rapha, the God who heals.

It is God's will to heal every time. Jesus was beaten for our healing (by His stripes we are healed). He is not getting beaten in heaven every time someone needs to be healed just like He is not getting crucified every time someone gets saved. Salvation and healing are finished works of Jesus Christ.

God is the healer. In Acts 10:34 it says God is no respecter of persons, which means he does not show favoritism. If God provided salvation for one, He provided for all. If He provided healing to one, He provided healing to all. The key is to accept by faith what Jesus has already done for us.

Some teach Paul's thorn in the flesh was a sickness or an eye disease and God would not heal him. Other types of wrong teachings include: God only heals spiritually not physically, healing passed away, or God heals some and not others.

Sometimes people misunderstand God's word, sometimes they elevate their personal experience on healing above God's word instead of letting God's word be the authority on healing. This always leads to doubt and unbelief.

Paul's thorn in 2 Corinthians is called "a messenger of Satan", not an illness. Paul never said that God would not heal Him or that God would not help him. Paul said that he sought the Lord three times and the Lord told him that His grace was sufficient and that the power of Christ would rest upon Him. Paul said, when he was weak, then through Christ he was made strong.

Jesus' grace is more than enough for any problem we face.

Also, in 2 Timothy 3:11, Paul comments he endured persecutions and afflictions, stating, "And out of them all the Lord delivered me."

When the bible talks about Paul's infirmity, the word infirmity in this case is translated as weakness in the Greek, not sickness as it is in some other scriptures. If we look at this situation rationally, the Lord certainly did not want Paul to go His entire life with a messenger from Satan tormenting him. Nor would the Lord want us to go through life with something from the devil, such as sickness, especially since Jesus already paid the price for it.

Jesus came to destroy the works of the devil (1 John 3:8), and God certainly doesn't want His people to live under the devil's bondage.

Acts 10:38 38 how God anointed Jesus of Nazareth with the Holy Spirit and with power, who went about doing good and healing all who were oppressed by the devil, for God was with Him.

Sickness and disease are an oppression by the devil as it says in Acts 10:38. God does not want us oppressed by the devil. Let's stop trying to justify our sickness and start magnifying the Lord. The Lord is bigger than any sickness or disease.

Mark 16:15-18 THE GREAT COMMISSION: 15 **And He said to them, "Go into all the world and preach the gospel to every creature. 16 He who believes and is baptized will be saved; but he who does not believe will be condemned. 17 And these signs will follow those who [a]believe: In My name they will cast out demons; they will speak with new tongues; 18 they[b] will take up serpents; and if they drink anything deadly, it will by no means hurt them; they will lay hands on the sick, and they will recover."**

As Christians, we must understand how the Kingdom of God works: by faith.

John 6:28-29 28 **Then they said to Him, "What shall we do, that we may work the works of God?" 29 Jesus answered and said to them, "This is the work of God, that you believe in Him whom He sent."**

CHAPTER 3

Hear, Believe and Receive

~

Romans 10:8-16 8 But what does it say? "The word is near you, in your mouth and in your heart" (that is, the word of faith which we preach): 9 that if you confess with your mouth the Lord Jesus and believe in your heart that God has raised Him from the dead, you will be saved. 10 For with the heart one believes unto righteousness, and with the mouth confession is made unto salvation. 11 For the Scripture says, "Whoever believes on Him will not be put to shame." 12 For there is no distinction between Jew and Greek, for the same Lord over all is rich to all who call upon Him. 13 For "whoever calls on the name of the Lord shall be saved."

14 How then shall they call on Him in whom they have not believed? And how shall they believe in Him of whom they have not heard? And how shall they hear without a preacher? 15 And how shall they preach unless they are sent? As it is written:

"How beautiful are the feet of those who [a]preach the gospel of peace,
Who bring glad tidings of good things!"

16 But they have not all obeyed the gospel. For Isaiah says, "Lord, who has believed our report?"

How do we obey the gospel? We obey by believing from the heart. Remember that the gospel is not just salvation, it includes healing and deliverance. Healing works the same way as salvation; we hear the message, believe the message and receive the promise. Jesus paid the price for it all. We need to see healing as a completed work just like salvation.

Sozo is the Greek word that translates salvation, saved, healed and delivered. Looking at the previous scriptures in Romans, replace the words saved or salvation with healed or healing. When reading it this way, we can bring healing alive. Start your healing from a place of victory, not as a victim. If we do not believe healing is a finished work, we will be striving to make it happen or trying to get God to do it. Healing is a finished work and it is ours. Jesus already provided for our healing, He is waiting for us to receive it.

How do we get healing to manifest? We do not need more information or facts, we don't need to sing more songs or quote more scriptures without having wisdom, knowledge and understanding. If we lack revelation, we are just repeating words. We need a revelation of God's truth, we need God's wisdom and understanding. God says if we lack wisdom to ask Him and He will give it.

Revelation is God revealing divine truth to us through the Holy Spirit. Facts are not beneficial when you need God results. Facts do not set you free. Truth alone does not set you free. Head knowledge is not the same as revelation knowledge. People can quote scriptures all day long without any change. It is the truth you know that sets you free. To get revelation from God, you must spend time with Him, meditating on His word. When we meditate on God's word, we are watering those seeds planted through the word so they can produce a harvest.

John 8:31-32 31 Then Jesus said to those Jews who believed Him, "If you abide in My word, you are My disciples indeed. 32 And you shall know the truth, and the truth shall make you free."

To get free from any situation, we need to abide in the word, knowing the truth. Be a disciple (a student of the word), not just a convert. It's the truth we know that sets us free. It's difficult to reap the benefits of something if you do not know it's yours. Remember, Jesus is the word. He is the way, the truth and the life. Jesus is healing.

CHAPTER 4

Our Thoughts Direct Our Life

~

Throughout the scriptures, Jesus talks about doubt, unbelief and fear. He also talks about having a hardened heart. Doubt is a feeling of uncertainty, distrust, or fear. Unbelief is skepticism, believing things are impossible. Fear is a tactic from the enemy to keep us from God's blessings. Our heart is the soil in which we plant God's word. A hard heart is difficult to penetrate.

2 Timothy 1:7 says that God has not given us a spirit of fear. Fear is not from God. When fear is present, we are not in faith. The devil will attempt to place thoughts and fears in our minds about how sick we are, how bad our disease is, he will tell us that we will never be well, we are going to die, our situation is too far gone, and on and on. The devil will try to get us to doubt the goodness of God. Even though the devil is a liar, we can receive these thoughts as truths and believe his lies. The devil can only get the upper hand through deception, fear and intimidation. He has no authority over us except what we allow through fear, doubt and unbelief. When we agree with the devil, we will get what he has for us.

We must meditate on God's word and gain revelation to overcome doubt, unbelief, fear and a hardened heart.

James 1:6-8 6 But let him ask in faith, with no doubting, for he who doubts is like a wave of the sea driven and tossed by the wind. 7 For let not that man suppose that he will receive anything from the Lord; 8 *he is* a double-minded man, unstable in all his ways.

The Lord says to ask in faith, with no doubting. Doubt blocks answered prayer.

Matthew 13:58 58 Now He did not do many mighty works there because of their unbelief.

Mark 6:5-6 5 Now He could do no mighty work there, except that He laid His hands on a few sick people and healed *them.* 6 And He marveled because of their unbelief. Then He went about the villages in a circuit, teaching.

Even Jesus could not do miracles because of the people's unbelief.

Mark 8:17 17 But Jesus, being aware of *it,* said to them, "Why do you reason because you have no bread? Do you not yet perceive nor understand? Is your heart [a]still hardened?

Hardness of heart is a condition that causes spiritual blindness. It stems from doubt and unbelief, thinking like the world instead of thinking like God. The hard heart dulls our ability to perceive and understand God's truths. Our hardness of heart causes a spiritual blindness and prevents us from receiving the promises of God.

Proverbs 23:7 7 **For as he thinks in his heart, so *is* he. "Eat and drink!" he says to you, But his heart is not with you.**

Proverbs 3:5 5 **Trust in the Lord with all your heart, And lean not on your own understanding;**

Paul's prayers are relevant to us today:

1. **Ephesians 1:17-20** We need the eyes of our hearts opened.

2. **Ephesians 3:16-20** We need to know the love of God. Ask God for a revelation of His love. A revelation of God's love will change you. A revelation of God's love will change the way you think and what you believe.

Matthew 13:18-23 18 "Therefore hear the parable of the sower: 19 **When anyone hears the word of the kingdom, and does not understand** *it,* **then the wicked** *one* **comes and snatches away what was sown in his heart. This is he who received seed by the wayside.** 20 **But he who received the seed on stony places, this is he who hears the word and immediately receives it with joy;** 21 **yet he has no root in himself, but endures only for a while. For when tribulation or persecution arises because of the word, immediately he stumbles.** 22 **Now he who received seed among the thorns is he who hears the word, and the cares of this world and the deceitfulness of riches choke the word, and he becomes unfruitful.** 23 **But he who received seed on the good ground is he who hears the word and understands** *it,* **who indeed bears fruit and produces: some a hundredfold, some sixty, some thirty."**

The ground or soil is your heart. The word of God pertaining to healing is the seed. We water the seed by meditating on the healing scriptures. We may need to hear the word of healing more than one time before it produces fruit.

Too many times we water the word of the sickness and hear over and over what the doctor says. We study our illness, meditating on what our problem is. To get healing to manifest, we must switch gears. We must hear the word of God over and over; we must hear the word of God more than the doctor. We must have more healing scriptures planted in our heart than medical knowledge. Whichever seed is watered will grow. Make sure it is the seed of healing.

Proverbs 4:23 23 **Keep your heart with all diligence, For out of it** *spring* **the issues of life.**

To prepare our hearts to receive God's benefits, we must meditate on His word. If you are reading this book, you may need to read it more than one time to get a revelation of the truth.

Proverbs 4:1-2 1 **Hear,** *my* **children, the instruction of a father, And give attention to know understanding;** 2 **For I give you good doctrine: Do not forsake my law.**

Proverbs 4:4-7 4 **He also taught me, and said to me: "Let your heart retain my words; Keep my commands, and live.** 5 **Get wisdom! Get understanding! Do not forget, nor turn away from the words of my mouth.** 6 **Do not forsake her, and she will preserve you; Love her, and she will keep you.** 7 **Wisdom** *is* **the principal thing;** *Therefore* **get wisdom. And in all your getting, get understanding.**

The Lord has instructions throughout the bible on how to have victory in every area of our lives. We have a part to play. Sometimes we choose not to follow God's instructions and at other times, we may be too lazy to find out what the instructions are. Being victorious does take some effort on our part. Sometimes we beg God to do something for us, and He has. Jesus gave us His authority and we need to use it. We must partake of the divine nature as it talks about in 2 Peter 1:3-11.

A couple of years ago, I had been working with a group of second graders on hand washing. I had a bottle of Glo Germ to simulate germs, a black box and a black light. The idea was to place a small amount of the Glo Germ on their hands, the kids would rub their hands together, then they would place their hands in the box and look at them under the black light to see how many germs they had before washing their hands.

Next, the children would wash their hands and look again under the black light to see how well they had washed their hands. As I was dispensing the Glo Germ onto the children's hands, the Glo Germ solution was running onto my hands. I kept rubbing the greasy solution into my hands. One little girl asked me to put my hands into the box. She looked into the box and then looked up at me with a look of shock and her eyes were wide open. She said, "Your hands don't glow!" I immediately looked at my hands in the box. My hands didn't glow! As I stood up, the Lord spoke to me saying, "Germs can't hurt you because you are a partaker of the divine nature."

This was a great reminder to me that God's word does not come to pass automatically. We have a part to play, we must partake in what the Lord has already provided.

Our thoughts are powerful. Where our thoughts take us, we follow. When the devil places thoughts in our minds, they are not our thoughts until we agree with them. Therefore, think only on good things.

CHAPTER 5

Perceptions

~

There can be a room full of people and each person's perception of the exact same event can be very different. Our perception of our circumstance will direct the outcome of the problem. If we see the problem as bigger than God, we will not get positive results.

In Numbers, The Lord told Moses to send men to spy out the land of Canaan which the Lord had prepared and promised to give to the children of Israel. When Joshua and Caleb returned from spying out the land, they had a good report and said even if there are giants in the land, we are well able to overcome them because the Lord is with us. Then the other men spoke up and said that the giants were stronger than the Israelites and they were like grasshoppers in their own sight. The Israelites even wanted to stone Joshua and Caleb for their good report.

How are you seeing your circumstance? How are you seeing yourself? Are you looking at your circumstance from your spiritual or your natural eyes?

1 Samuel 17 is the story of David and Goliath. The Israelites had been tormented for 40 days by Goliath and the Philistine army. None of the Israelites would dare to challenge Goliath due to fearing him. When David came along, he had a completely different view of the situation. First, he knew who his God was. Second, he knew who he was and thirdly he knew who his enemy was. His enemy was an uncircumcised Philistine who was not in a covenant relationship with God. David came boldly before Goliath. He came in the name of the Lord and defeated Goliath with one stone and Goliath's own sword.

2 Kings 6 Elisha prayed that his servant's eyes be opened so he could see that those with them were more than those that were with the enemy.

How we see ourselves in the circumstance matters. If we see ourselves as defeated, we will be. But, if we can see our circumstance as God sees, we will be victorious. We must be able to envision ourselves well, without sickness; envision ourselves whole and healed. Magnify the Lord, not the problem. Whatever we are magnifying becomes bigger.

I am not suggesting eliminating physicians, but suggesting assessing where we have placed our faith, in God or man.

CHAPTER 6

How to Be an Overcomer

~

2 Corinthians 10:4-5 4 For the weapons of our warfare *are* not [a]carnal but mighty in God for pulling down strongholds, 5 casting down arguments and every high thing that exalts itself against the knowledge of God, bringing every thought into captivity to the obedience of Christ,

The Lord tells us to take our thoughts captive and make them obey His word. We must renew our minds. We cannot elevate medical knowledge above God's word and be victorious.

Romans 12:2 (NLT): 2 Don't copy the behavior and customs of this world, but let God transform you into a new person by changing the way you think. Then you will learn to know God's will for you, which is good and pleasing and perfect.

Notice God wants to change our thinking, not our behaviors. As our thinking and believing begins to line up with God's thinking and His way of doing things, our body will align with the word of God. We will be transformed. When we agree with God's truths, we begin to get God's results.

We live in the world but are not of the world. Our home is heaven. As Christians, we do not need to submit to the world's way of thinking and their way of doing things. If we want God's results, we must do things His way. We cannot put God in a box; we cannot do things our own way; we cannot doubt His word and expect His answers. The bible says that man's traditions, in other words, man's way of doing things, make God's word ineffective (Mark 7:13).

God's ways are higher than our ways and His thoughts are higher than our thoughts. His ways don't always make sense to the world; for example: If you're broke, God says give and it shall be given unto you. God's way is always the right way.

The difference between someone getting their prayer answered and the person who doesn't get their prayer answered, is what and who they believe. The difference is who we are agreeing with; God, sickness, our body, our feelings or the devil. It is that simple. It is imperative we agree with God.

CHAPTER 7

Spirit, Soul and Body

~

SPIRIT: Once we are born again, we have everything we will ever need living on the inside of us. Our Spirit is perfect and we have all spiritual blessings. All answers to prayer reside within us. Healing lives in us, resurrection power lives in us. We just need to let it out.

SOUL: Our soul consists of our emotions, our will, it is our heart; it's where we believe and receive. Our soul is the key to answered prayer. The soul is the filter/receiver to get things from the spirit realm into the physical realm. If our soul is blocked with unbelief it will be difficult to get healing from the spiritual realm into the physical world. Life happens and causes our filters to become clogged at times. Unbelief, doubt, fears, past abuses, unforgiveness, offenses, wrong teachings and man's traditions are some of the things that will "clog" our filters. To clean our filter, we must renew our minds with the word of God.

BODY: We have a body, which houses our spirit and our soul. Some bodies have sickness or pain. For sickness or pain to leave our physical bodies, we need to get our soul and spirit to agree.

There is power in agreement. Our spirit says we are healed, but if our soul agrees with our broken body, we will not see healing manifest. But if our soul agrees with our spirit, our body has no choice but to be well.

The soul is the key to what we have or do not have in life. God has given us free will and He will never override our will. We have the choice to believe God's word or not.

When sickness comes on a person and that person visits the doctor, the doctor gives them the medical outlook on the situation. Many Christians spend more time meditating on what the doctor says than on what God says. Looking things up on the internet and studying the disease is not helpful if we are looking to be healed. Whatever we ponder, meditate on or study, our hearts will become softened to. Whatever we neglect to meditate on, our heart becomes hardened to.

My daughter called me on a Friday as I was driving to work. She called for prayer, informing me she was 21 weeks pregnant and the doctor had found a large mass that put her at risk for bleeding and the baby at risk for not developing properly. She said she had to see the specialist because she was considered a high-risk pregnancy.

I gave my daughter a few instructions. First, I gave her some scriptures that came to mind, told her to look them up, and meditate on them. I also told her to stay off the internet and not to study what the doctor had told her. I informed her I would drive down to her home on Saturday.

Saturday, we spent about 4 hours going over healing scriptures and watched a healing testimony to encourage her. At the end, I prayed for her (less than 1 minute). My daughter said she was at complete peace and knew that everything would be alright.

The following Friday, she went for her appointment with the specialist. The specialist was taking a long time completing the ultrasound and asked, "Where did the doctor see this mass?" Then the specialist said the mass was gone, the baby was fine, my daughter was fine and there was no need to come back! Praise the Lord!

The Lord is so good! After my daughter had told me the praise report, the Lord told me he did not do anything, but that my daughter had just received what He had already done 2000 years ago.

If we can see that healing is a finished work, it is much easier to get healing to manifest. If we are trying to get God to do something, it is more difficult than just receiving what He has already been provided. We don't have to convince God to heal us, He already did.

CHAPTER 8

Faith and Unbelief

~

1 John 5:4 4 For whatever is born of God overcomes the world. And this is the victory that has overcome the world—[a]our faith.

Romans 10:17 17 So then faith *comes* by hearing, and hearing by the word of God.

Hebrews 11:1 11 Now faith is the [a]substance of things hoped for, the [b]evidence of things not seen.

We do not need faith for things we already have in our possession but that's how a lot of people look at healing. They will believe they are healed when they can physically feel it or see it. They accept what the doctor says and look at how they feel to determine if they are healed or not. They won't believe it until they see it. That is not faith. We need to stand on what God's word says no matter how we feel or what we see. And God says that we are healed by the stripes of Jesus. Faith is the evidence of things not seen. Faith is believing God no matter what. Faith is standing firm on the promises of Jesus.

Hebrews 11:6 6 But without faith *it is* impossible to please *Him,* for he who comes to God must believe that He is, and *that* He is a rewarder of those who diligently seek Him.

Faith comes by hearing God's word and doubt comes from hearing reports contrary to God's word. We need faith to receive from God. God says He is a rewarder of those who diligently seek Him, not diligently seek the doctor's advice. (I work with doctors and have nothing against them, just making a point).

Hebrews 10:23 23 Let us hold fast the confession of our hope without wavering, for He who promised is faithful.

What confession are we making? Are we holding fast to our confession without wavering? Is it a confession of faith in God's word or a confession of how big and tough the disease is? How the disease is hereditary and there is nothing we can do? How deadly the doctor's report is?

Isaiah 54:17 No weapon formed against you shall prosper.

We must see sickness as a weapon formed against us and fight it. Stand against sickness. Tell sickness, "No! Sickness, you will not prosper! I am a child of God and healing is mine!"

The bible says out of the abundance of a man's heart, he speaks. If you have more of the doctor's report coming out of your mouth than the word of God, you need to renew your mind to get God's word flowing from your mouth. If you don't have an abundance of God's word coming out, at least shut your mouth so the word of the doctor/disease is not coming out. The bible says we have what we say.

We have all been given the measure of faith. If you have Jesus living in you, you have His faith and Jesus' faith has never failed. If you don't have Jesus, you will seriously want to make a decision for Him sooner than later.

1 John 4:17 17 Love has been perfected among us in this: that we may have boldness in the day of judgement; because as He is, so are we in this world.

The previous verse says we are just like Jesus in this world. We have what He says we have, and we are who He says we are. We are more than conquerors. Christ means the Anointed One. This means we have the healing anointing in us if Christ dwells in us.

Now that we understand we need faith for our promises to manifest, we need to discuss the enemy of our faith, unbelief. Any time you have unbelief mixed with your faith, you will not see answered prayer.

I have children and have experienced injured and sick kids and grandchildren. Yes, I have been known to take them to the doctor. I am also a Registered Nurse and sometimes think like a nurse. I can tell you that when I respond to a situation in the name of Jesus, instead of like a nurse or a parent, I have gotten better, quicker results. I wish I could say I respond boldly in Jesus name every time, but I cannot. Anytime we have any doubts about healing, we better make sure we do all we can for the child including medical attention.

To stop us from responding in the name of Jesus, the enemy is usually right there whispering in our ears to instill fear. What better way to instill fear than to attack our children. The devil has no problems attacking children with sickness and disease. He is our enemy. When children become sick and they are not old enough to understand God's word, the parents are responsible to believe for the child's healing. This is not meant to place blame or condemnation on anyone.

God has provided the healing and given us His authority. The believing for healing is up to us. The commanding the sickness to leave is up to us. The responding in faith is up to us. Get mad at the enemy and take back your child's health.

In Mark 9, a father brought his son to Jesus to be healed because the disciples could not heal him. The father of the boy said to Jesus, "If you can do anything." Jesus said, "If you can believe, all things are possible to those who believe." The father responded, "Lord, I believe; help my unbelief."

We are believers, but sometimes we need help with our unbelief especially when it is our child that is facing sickness. The disciples later asked Jesus why they couldn't cast it out of the boy. Jesus had said that this kind, meaning this kind of unbelief, only comes out by prayer and fasting. We must get rid of unbelief.

When we see our child or a loved one sick and helpless, this can bring doubt and worry. To overcome the doubt, we need to renew our mind. If we are up against a serious illness, we cannot let anything in but God's healing word. We cannot look at the physical circumstance as greater than God's word. Remember, Satan likes to do a lot of roaring but that's all it is, a lot of noise.

Some years ago, I had a patient that had a swollen right arm. I asked if he wanted me to pray for him. He excitedly said, "Yes!" I prayed the prayer of faith, commanded swelling to go and commanded his arm to be healed and left the room.

The next day, I went back to check on him in the morning. To my surprise, his arm was twice as big as the day before. I was mortified. I said, "Those aren't the results I was looking for." He replied, "Me either."

I didn't know what else to even say to this poor man and I was feeling personally responsible for his enormous arm. I was embarrassed to say the least and I never offered to pray for him again, not that he would have wanted me to with the results I was getting.

This patient happened to have an appointment to get his arm checked this same day. When he returned from the appointment, I immediately grabbed his paperwork. His diagnosis was pseudogout. This is a real diagnosis, but what caught my attention was the "pseudo" part of the diagnosis. Pseudo means: not genuine, false or a sham. All I could think was that the devil roared and I fell for it. I was looking at the circumstances and it made me doubt the healing. But I was ready the next time the devil roared.

About a week later, my son looked like he had pink eye in one eye. We prayed for him and the next morning, it was in both eyes and looked much worse. My husband told him to go wash his eyes, look in the mirror and command the pink eye to go! My son did and it was gone by the next day.

Right after my son was healed, we went to stay with my oldest daughter and grandkids for a few days. While there, my five-year-old daughter developed pink eye. Now I was angry at the devil. I took my daughter into the bathroom where the window was open and loudly shouted at pink eye to go in Jesus' name! My oldest daughter yelled at me, "Keep it down, I have neighbors!" I didn't care. I wasn't dealing with pink eye.

The next day, my daughter woke up with no more signs of pink eye. Pink eye was gone. Now, if you are wondering if it really was pink eye, the answer is yes. After we left, my grandkids developed pink eye and my daughter took them to the doctor for eye drops.

The Lord's word does not automatically come to pass. The bible is full of God's promises. If we are not meditating on the word of the Lord, we can miss our blessing. Satan does not play fair and attempts to get us to buy into his lies. The only way he can beat us is through deception.

When we are facing terrible circumstances, we cannot be giving the circumstance our full attention. We cannot waiver from the word of the Lord. We should never have plan B in place, "just in case." Stick to plan A. Stay single-minded. The Lord tells us to stand firm on His word and then keep standing. Whatever gets the most of our attention, wins. In order to see healing, our entire focus must be the prize, not the what ifs. Magnify God, not the problem.

It is not wise to wait until you are face to face with a horrible circumstance before you put your faith into action. For instance, don't wait until a life-threatening illness comes into your life before you study the scriptures. Practice rebuking headaches, colds and pains now. Faith without works is dead faith.

The more positive results you see as you begin to exercise your faith, the more confident you become. Doubt and unbelief come exactly the same way faith does, by hearing. The difference is who you are hearing. Faith comes by hearing God and unbelief by hearing the enemy.

James 1:5-8 5 If any of you lacks wisdom, let him ask of God, who gives to all liberally and without reproach, and it will be given to him. 6 But let him ask in faith, with no doubting, for he who doubts is like a wave of the sea driven and tossed by the wind. 7 For let not that man suppose that he will receive anything from the Lord; 8 *he is* a double-minded man, unstable in all his ways.

When we have faith and doubt working together, the doubt cancels our prayer of faith. Being double-minded is like being two-souled, our heart is wavering between belief and unbelief; we are believing two things contrary to each other and have not set our mind (heart) fully on God's promise. We must believe with our whole heart, if not, God says we should not expect anything.

Mark 5: 22-24 22 And behold, one of the rulers of the synagogue came, Jairus by name. And when he saw Him, he fell at His feet 23 and begged Him earnestly,

saying, "My little daughter lies at the point of death. Come and lay Your hands on her, that she may be healed, and she will live." 24 So *Jesus* went with him, and a great multitude followed Him and thronged Him.

Mark 5:35-42 35 While He was still speaking, *some* came from the ruler of the synagogue's *house* who said, "Your daughter is dead. Why trouble the Teacher any further?"

36 As soon as Jesus heard the word that was spoken, He said to the ruler of the synagogue, "Do not be afraid; only believe." 37 And He permitted no one to follow Him except Peter, James, and John the brother of James. 38 Then He came to the house of the ruler of the synagogue, and saw [a]a tumult and those who wept and wailed loudly. 39 When He came in, He said to them, "Why make this commotion and weep? The child is not dead, but sleeping."

40 And they ridiculed Him. But when He had put them all outside, He took the father and the mother of the child, and those *who were* with Him, and entered where the child was lying. 41 Then He took the child by the hand, and said to her, "Talitha, cumi," which is translated, "Little girl, I say to you, arise." 42 Immediately the girl arose and walked, for she was twelve years *of age.* And they were overcome with great amazement.

When the word came that Jairus' daughter died, Jesus told him not to fear and to **only** believe. He put the crowd of unbelief outside. Jesus never broke a sweat over sickness or death. He just spoke to it. Jesus made it simple. He said speak to your mountain (problem).

My father-in-law passed away several years ago. When he died, my husband just commanded the death spirit to leave in Jesus name and spoke life to his dad. Within a few minutes his dad was back. That's how easy raising the dead is. No sweat.

We hear things like, "She was believing for healing, she was so faithful, and she died." or we question why the Lord didn't heal her? Healing has nothing to do with our faithfulness, it has everything to do with God's faithfulness. God is faithful, but do we believe God?

Unbelief is the enemy of our faith. When we need healing, we need to diligently seek God. God said that He is a rewarder of those who diligently seek Him. Sometimes, we think it's God's fault when we do not get our prayers answered. All of God's promises in His word are yes and amen. It is never God's fault if we miss His promises; it is our responsibility to know the word and use our authority. There is good news in this, it means we can do something about unanswered prayer. It's much better than thinking maybe God will or maybe He won't answer my prayer; or you just never know what God is going to do. It's difficult to be in faith if you don't know what to expect.

God has given us His word and His authority, so we can be victorious in every area of our life. God has provided salvation for all and the same is true about healing. Healing is available to all. Not everyone is saved and not everyone gets healed. A preacher preaches on salvation and some but not all get saved. The same thing happens when someone preaches on healing, some get healed and some don't. The difference is the person listening, (the hearer of the word) do they believe the message? People who believe the message respond to the message in faith.

Some causes of doubt and unbelief: Wrong teaching, wrong thinking, lack of understanding, lack knowledge, fear, unforgiveness, etc. will block our answers to prayer and God's blessings.

When our heart is wavering between faith and doubt, we will not have answered prayer. Our heart is our soul, our will, and understanding of God's word. God has given us free will and will not override our will. God cannot override our belief system. God has done His part by providing healing. Believing and receiving is the believer's part. We can completely change the way we think by renewing our minds through the word of God.

We don't need more faith, just less doubt and unbelief.

CHAPTER 9
Final Thoughts

~

Psalm 18:30 30 **As for God, His way is perfect; the word of the Lord is proven; He is a shield to all who trust in Him.**

Job 22:28 28 **You will also declare a thing, and it will be established for you; so light will shine on your ways.**

We make a lot of declarations each day. We need to ensure they are in agreement with God. There are spiritual laws and Satan is very legalistic. If we are declaring negative words, the devil is happy to give us what we say.

Matthew 18:19 19 **"Again I say to you that if two of you agree on earth concerning anything that they ask, it will be done for them by My Father in Heaven. For where two or three are gathered together in My name, I am there in the midst of them."**

We need to agree with God, not sickness. We need other believers to get in agreement with us. Do not get in agreement with someone that just feels bad for you and will only pity you. Feeling badly or pitying someone will not get them healed. Don't look for coddling, look for deliverance from the situation. Look for someone that will agree with you and God. Look for someone that will tell you the truth. The truth you know will set you free. Keep unbelief away from the situation, put unbelief outside.

Matthew 9:29 29 **Then He touched their eyes, saying, "According to your faith let it be to you."**

Fear and faith work the same. Faith draws God. Fear draws in the enemy and he is happy to give you whatever you are fearing. Make sure you are in faith, not fear.

Matthew 7:7-8 7 **"Ask and it will be given to you; seek and you will find; knock and the door will be opened to you.** 8 **For everyone who asks receives; the one who seeks finds; and to the one who knocks, the door will be opened.**

Seek healing, not sickness.

Philippians 4:8-9 8 **Finally, brethren, whatever things are true, whatever things are noble, whatever things are just, whatever things are pure, whatever things are lovely, whatever things are of good report, if there is any virtue and if there is anything praiseworthy – meditate on these things.** 9 **The thing which you learned and received and heard and saw in me, these do, and the God of peace will be with you.**

God tells us to think or meditate on good things.

Mark 9:23 23 **Jesus said to Him, "If you can believe, all things are possible to him who believes."**

All things are possible if we believe God. All means all.

Matthew 21:21-22 21 **So Jesus answered and said to them, "Assuredly, I say to you, if you have faith and do not doubt, you will not only do what was done to the fig tree, but also if you say to this mountain, 'Be removed and be cast into the sea,' it will be done.** 22 **And whatever things you ask in prayer, believing, you will receive."**

There is a difference between speaking to our mountain and speaking about our mountain. When we speak about the mountain, we are coming into agreement with it. When we are speaking to the mountain, we command it to move.

Examples:
1. I have a terrible headache and a stomach ache. I feel terrible. In fact, I am going to call into work. I must be coming down with something.

2. I command you, headache, to leave in the name of Jesus! Stomach ache go! In Jesus name! Thank you, Jesus!

Healing is that simple. If you command a symptom to leave and you feel no relief, do it again if you feel the need. Just know it is done. Practice, practice and practice again. And remember, it is not what you feel or see that matters, it's who and what you believe.

James 4:7 7 Therefore submit to God. Resist the devil and he will flee from you.

To submit to God is to trust Him, to trust His word no matter what we see. Submitting is yielding to His authority; God's will and our will are in agreement. When we are trusting God, we are standing with an unshakeable faith. When we submit to God, we stop leaning on our own understanding and rest in what the Lord has done. We do not want to submit to the sickness and let the sickness direct the situation.

To resist the devil is to deny his right to take what belongs to us, such as our health. To resist the devil is to resist sickness. This may impact our thinking: if we agree with sickness or fear, our will is aligned with the devil's will. That is not a place we want to be.

Faith will withstand the devil's actions or effects of his actions every time. Remember it says to resist the devil, not assist the devil. Speak life giving words. The devil knows who we are, he just hopes we don't know the power that resides in us as believers.

James 1:22-25 22 But be doers of the word, and not hearers only, deceiving yourselves. 23 For if anyone is a hearer of the word and not a doer, he is like a man observing his natural face in a mirror; 24 for he observes himself, goes away, and immediately forgets what kind of man he was. 25 But he who looks into the perfect law of liberty and continues *in it,* and is not a forgetful hearer but a doer of the work, this one will be blessed in what he does.

James 2:18-24 18 But someone will say, "You have faith, and I have works." Show me your faith without [a]your works, and I will show you my faith by [b]my works. 19 You believe that there is one God. You do well. Even the demons believe—and tremble! 20 But do you want to know, O foolish man, that faith without works is [c]dead? 21 Was not Abraham our father justified by works when he offered Isaac his son on the altar? 22 Do you see that faith was working together with his works, and by works faith was made [d]perfect? 23 And the Scripture was fulfilled which says, "Abraham believed God, and it was [e]accounted to him for righteousness." And he was called the friend of God. 24 You see then that a man is justified by works, and not by faith only.

It never does anyone any good to hear the gospel and never receive Jesus or never confess Him as Lord. In churches all over, people believe in Jesus, but there is more than just believing that He exists. James says that even the demons believe. We must put our faith into action and get born again. (See the front of the book).

The Lord says we must put our faith into action, or we are deceiving ourselves. It's not even the devil deceiving us, we are deceiving ourselves. We quote scriptures and sing songs about who we are in Christ, the victory we have in Christ, we sing songs about a defeated devil, and yet, sometimes we live like we are powerless to the circumstances that arise in our lives.

Faith in action, is doing the word. If someone truly believes the gospel, they will invite Jesus to be their Lord and Savior. When we truly believe what we say, we will act on it.

When we are believing for healing, we will stop talking about the problem and start confessing the answer; we will try to do something we couldn't do before; we will resist the sickness, we will study the scriptures. We will praise God before we ever see the manifestation.

Hebrews 4:1-3 1 Therefore, since a promise remains of entering His rest, let us fear lest any of you seem to have come short of it. 2 For indeed the gospel was preached to us as well as to them; but the word which they heard did not profit them, [a]not being mixed with faith in those who heard *it*. 3 For we who have believed do enter that rest, as He has said:

> "So I swore in My wrath,
> 'They shall not enter My rest,' "

although the works were finished from the foundation of the world.

Hebrews 4:6-7 6 Since therefore it remains that some *must* enter it, and those to whom it was first preached did not enter because of disobedience, 7 again He designates a certain day, saying in David, "Today," after such a long time, as it has been said:

> "Today, if you will hear His voice,
> Do not harden your hearts."

We DO NOT need to strive to get God to do things for us, we only need to rest in what He has already done. The Israelites never entered the promised land until the unbelieving, grumbling, complaining generation died off.

Ephesians 3:20 20 Now to Him who is able to do exceedingly abundantly above all that we ask or think, according to the power that works in us.

We can have exceedingly abundantly above all that we ask or think, according to the power that works in us. Did you hear that? According to the power that works in us. It is up to us.

Jesus tells us that the power is working in us. We are not fighting a losing battle. Jesus won the war when he came out of the grave. He has given each and every one of us the same authority that He operated in while He was on the earth. We need to take our stand from a point of victory, not from the point of a victim. We are more than conquerors. Jesus' faith never fails.

Last thoughts: Yes, Jesus did make doctors, but He never sent anyone to a doctor or psychiatrist. His power, the same power He entrusted to us, took care of everything. When we are treated by doctors, many times only the symptoms are treated by the medication and many times the side effects of the medication are as bad or worse than the actual illness. Jesus' way of doing things removes the mountain completely, removing sickness at the roots. Never stop taking your medication without a revelation from God. Start with praying against side effects. Again, I'm not against doctors, just making a point.

Today, there are a lot of sick Christians that do not know how to get healed. Many are in every healing line they can find with the same results every time, no change. I believe there is a time coming very soon that we, as the Church, are going to rise up and take what's rightfully ours. We will no longer put up with just getting by. We will no longer be as sick as the rest of the world, we will be their answer.

We are Jesus' voice on the earth, we are His hands and feet. We need to take Jesus at His word. We are believers and believers are supposed to believe. So, let's encourage one another in the Lord!

Remember, we have what we say. Start declaring your victory. Start praying for others. Start seeing results. Declare you are healed. Declare when you pray for others, they are healed. Healing is easy once you see things God's way.

HINT: If you are baptized in the Holy Spirit and speak in other tongues, do this often. Praying in the Spirit improves your immune system and brings revelation.

If you are not baptized in the Holy Spirit, I recommend getting "Wind Talkers: The Baptism of The Holy Spirit" by David Hallam. His book is available on Amazon and is, in my opinion, the best explanation of speaking in tongues and easily leads you through the process of receiving the gift. Otherwise, just ask God. ●

FINAL DECLARATION:
Psalm 118:17 I shall not die, but live, and declare the works of the Lord.